The ABC's of Surviving Cancer:

Alive, Beautiful, & Courageous

Tammy Trover

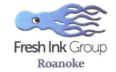

Fresh Ink Group
Roanoke

The ABC's of Surviving Cancer
Alive, Beautiful, & Courageous

Copyright © 2016
by Tammy Trover
All rights reserved

Fresh Ink Group
An Imprint of:
The Fresh Ink Group, LLC
PO Box 525
Roanoke, TX 76262
Email: info@FreshInkGroup.com
www.FreshInkGroup.com

Edition 1.0   2016

Book design by Ann Stewart / Fresh Ink Group

Cover & Editing by Stephen Geez / Fresh Ink Group

Artwork by Anik / Fresh Ink Group

Art Inspired by Robbie Howard

BISAC Subject Headings:
JNF024020 JUVENILE NONFICTION / Health & Daily Living / Diseases, Illnesses & Injuries
JNF024000 JUVENILE NONFICTION / Health & Daily Living / General
JNF008000 JUVENILE NONFICTION / Body, Mind & Spirit

Paper-cover ISBN-13: 978-1-936442-39-3
Hardcover ISBN-13: 978-1-936442-40-9
Ebook ISBN-13: 978-1-936442-41-6

The ABC's of Surviving Cancer:

Alive, Beautiful, & Courageous

Dedication

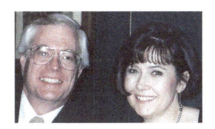

Brian and Darlene Pieper

For Brian and Darlene Pieper, who made my family theirs as we struggled together to beat my cancer. I don't know how I could have done all this without your love and support and constant help in every aspect of surviving.

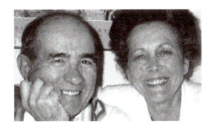

Armand and Nomi Carabello

To the memory of Armand and Nomi Carabello, honorary grandparents for my kids, a couple of wonderful souls who stood beside us and never let us want for anything.

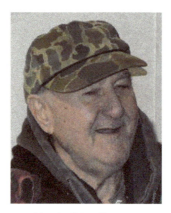

Uncle Bim Howard

To the memory of my Uncle Bim Howard, who bravely fought cancer until he could no more. You were my inspiration, one who has always been **there** for me.

Finally, for all the kids and their families facing such a difficult journey. If you remember to love each other like my friends and family love me, you'll accomplish more than you could ever imagine.

For more information about the cancer fight, visit the
American Cancer Society
at www.cancer.org
or call 1 (800) 227-2345.

Please share this story with family and friends.

If YOU have a brief but heartfelt story about your own fight with cancer, or someone you know fighting cancer, please attach it and a photo through the www.TammyTrover.com CONTACT page. I will share some of these with visitors to my website.

Please spread the word, post reviews at online bookstores, and tell me what you think through the website.

Thanks to all of you for your love and support!

Tammy Trover

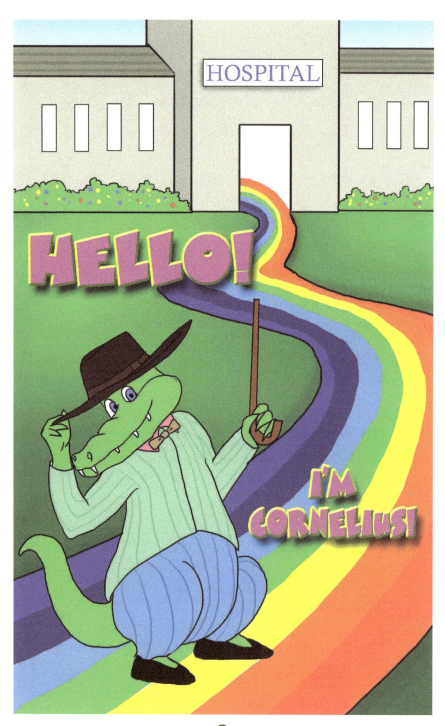

Cornelius is our cancer fighter.
He helps fight cancer
and make our days brighter.
He's here to guide you through this book
and help you laugh, as you learn and look.

Cornelius knows the fight ahead.
He'll brighten your days as you sleep in bed.
It's his job to help you know
you're never alone wherever you go.

Cornelius will guide and show you, too,
the things inside you, you never knew,
the things inside that keep you alive,
the things inside that help you survive.

He'll teach you things to help you cope,
things inside that give courage and hope.
Remember, it's his job; he knows what to do,
so let's fight the fire of cancer in you!

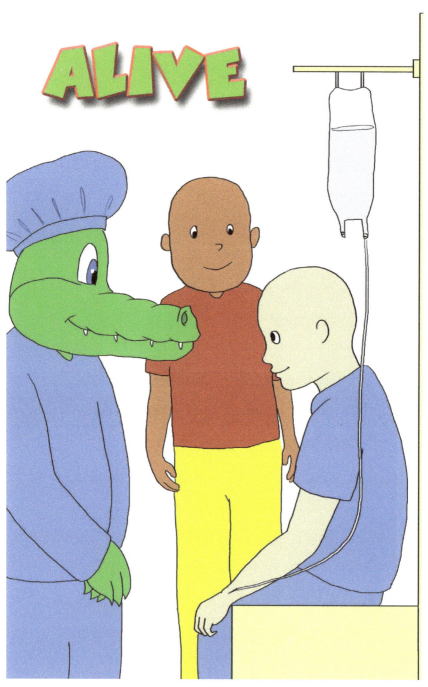

ALIVE

The ABC's of Surviving Cancer

"**A**" is for alive,
that's what I am.
This is my story and how it began.
When cancer came in,
it changed my days,
changed my thoughts
and changed my ways.

I often wonder what people see
when I see them staring at me.
I've lost my hair, can't eat at all.
I'm tiny and pale and very small.

Cancer doesn't care
if you're big or small,
short and fat, or skinny and tall.
It doesn't care
if you're happy or sad.
It doesn't care
if you're good or bad.

It doesn't matter where you live,
how much you love,
or what you give.
It affects us all, I hope you see,
big and small, you and me.

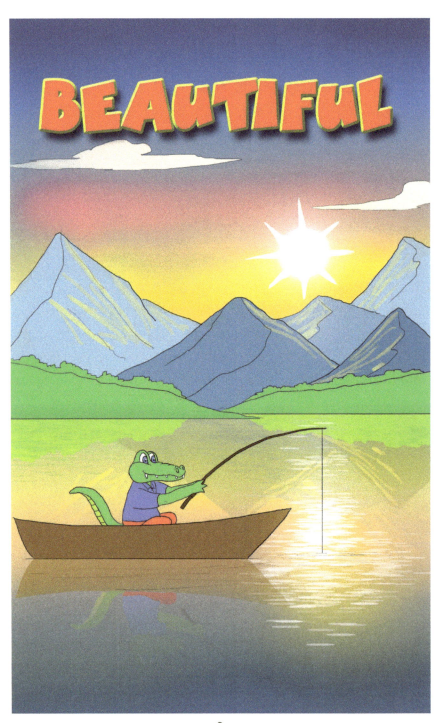

"B" is for beautiful
and the love we give,
not what you see, but how we live.
It doesn't describe my appearance,
you see;
it describes my heart
and what's inside me.

Beautiful is a small child's laugh,
a giggle at play while taking a bath.
Beautiful is what I want to remember,
a rainbow's colors,
a holiday in December.

Beautiful is something
cancer can't take.
It's the rise of the sun
or a boat on a lake.
It's in my heart, and it's in my head,
something to be felt, not just to be said.

Beauty can make us stronger, you see.
It makes us feel good, being you and me,
so no matter what happens,
remember my smile,
my beauty within,
my strength and my style.

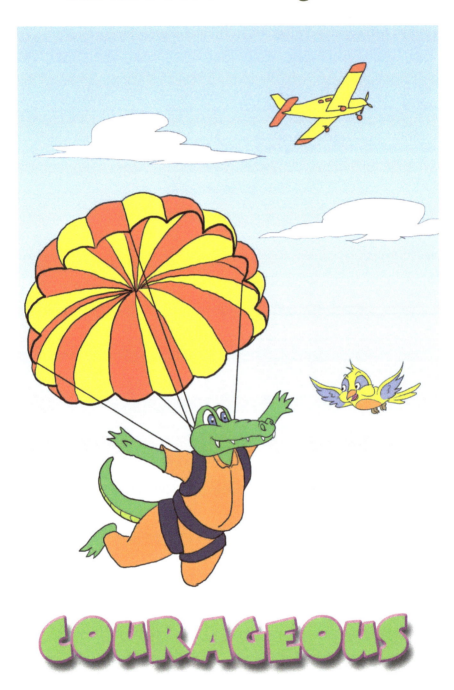

COURAGEOUS

"C" is for courageous; it's what we are,
jumping from a plane or wishing on a star.
Courageous is another
that cancer can't take.
Courage is something
that cancer can't break.

Courage is something
that begins in the heart.
It grows and it builds,
and it gives us a start.
It's something that God gave
to help in the fight.
It's a strength and a feeling
that turns darkness to light.

Courage is something that cannot be broken.
It's something we feel,
not something that's spoken.
It's something that's helped
by Mom and by Dad,
and something that helps
when we're happy or sad.

Courage is something
for the big and the small.
Courage is something for one and for all,
and no matter the outcome,
this struggle, you see,
courage is something that lives inside me.

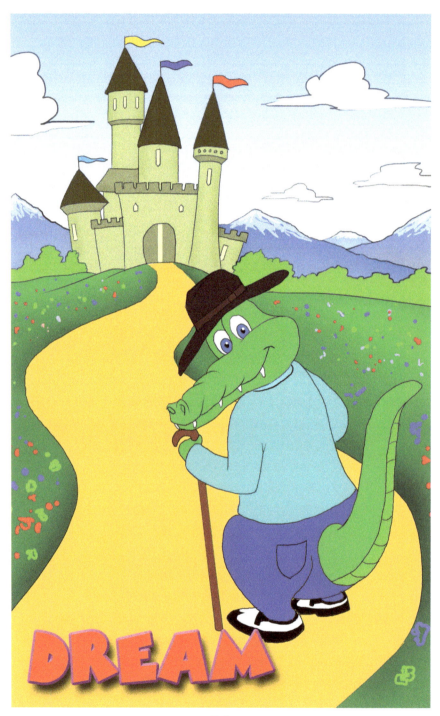

"D" is for dream,
whether by day or by night.
It helps us find hope
while we're fighting the fight.
Dreams bring life
to what starts in the mind,
so let's dream together
and see what we find.

What makes you dream?
Is it something you see?
Something you feel, or what you can be?
What makes you happy?
What makes you dream?
Is it time with a friend,
or chocolate ice cream?

Is it running or playing out in the park?
Is it toys in your room or a movie at dark?
Is it something we want
to be when we're all grown?
Or is it something we want
to do all on our own?

There are so many things
we imagine and dream,
like being a princess, a king, or a queen,
so if we can see, dream,
and know that it's true;
then the sky is the limit on what we can do.

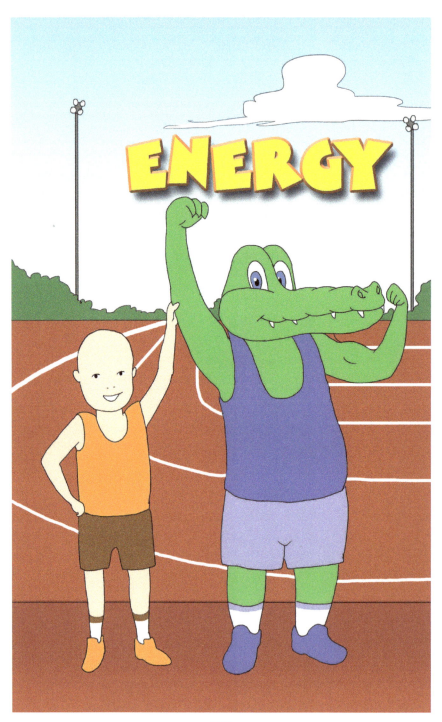

"E" is for energy and what gets me through
when I'm weak and I'm sick
and not sure what to do.
It does not come from a wall outlet, you see.
It comes from a place deep inside of me.

It's that thing that helps me get up when I fall,
and also what helps me
stand straight and stand tall.
Energy doesn't let me droop or stay down.
It helps me smile instead of wearing a frown.

Energy is something people definitely see
when they're chasing me around
and can't seem to catch me.
When I'm playing, laughing, and joking, too,
it's my energy that helps get me through.

So let's play, laugh, and have fun tonight.
Then Cornelius and I will continue the fight.
Remember, this energy stored up in me
will help in the fight; just wait and see.

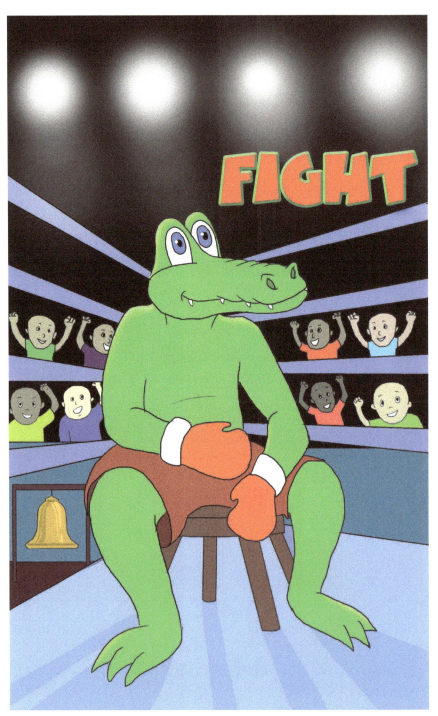

"F" is for fight
and what I do when I'm sick:
I carry on, I cry, I scream, and I kick.
But then I remember I'm never alone,
so I settle down, and I pick up the phone.

I call Cornelius, my family, and friends.
They'll help get me through
again and again.
They'll always be here to help in the fight.
They'll always be here,
turning darkness to light.

So no matter the battle
or pain I go through,
they're always here;
they know what to do.
They know I just need
to laugh and to smile
or just to sit and to hang out for a while.

They know that my days
can be up or be down,
and that I can't help it
when I still have to frown;
but they know that I'll never
give up the fight
'cause I know the future's
beautiful and bright.

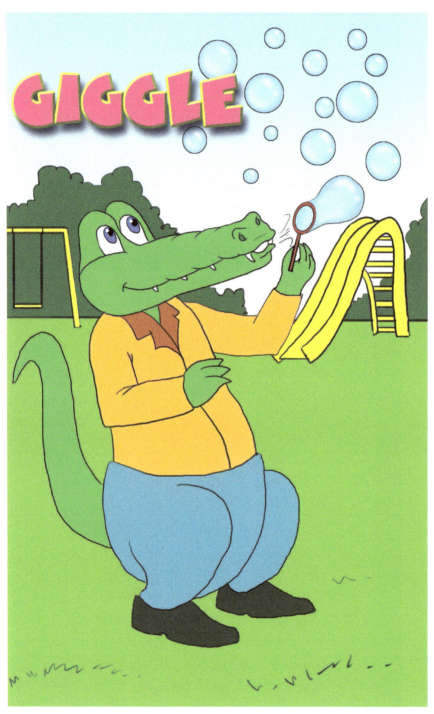

"G" is for giggle; it bubbles inside,
then has to come out
with nowhere to hide.
The way it feels
is completely outrageous,
and there is no doubt
it's completely contagious.

Once I get started, I can't seem to stop,
and I giggle so hard I feel like I'll pop.
Sometimes it slips out
when I least expect it,
and it happens when life
is crazy and hectic.

It might start from something
I see or I hear.
It might be from watching a movie I fear.
It might be because I have nothing to do,
Or it might slip out
when I hear someone scream, "Boo!"

It might be something to heal a bad day.
It might start with something
I do or I say,
and no matter how the giggle comes out,
it's definitely what's needed
to cure a good pout!

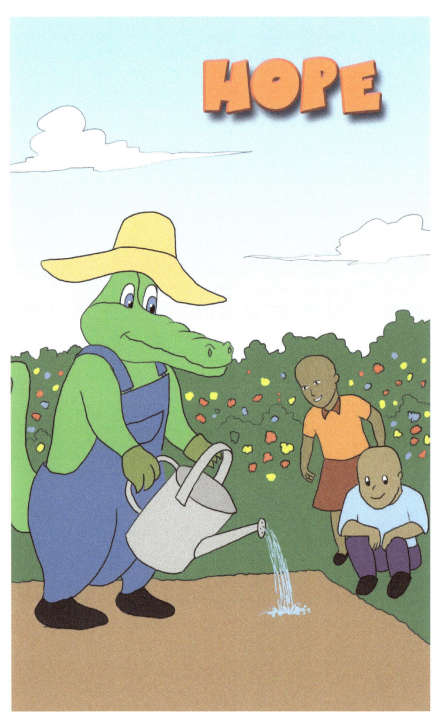

"**H**" is for hope, not something I see,
but something I feel that lives inside me.
Hope is something
you feel when I giggle.
It's something you feel
when I laugh and I wiggle.

See, although I may be smaller than you,
you taught me well, I know what to do.
Hope is something that I'll never lose.
It's something I feel
and something I choose.

It's something that helps me
always stay strong,
and something that helps
when the days grow long.
It's something I need
to help in the fight.
It's something inside
that stays out of sight.

Remember you helped put inside of me
so many things that no one can see,
things like beauty, love, and hope,
things like memories that help me cope.

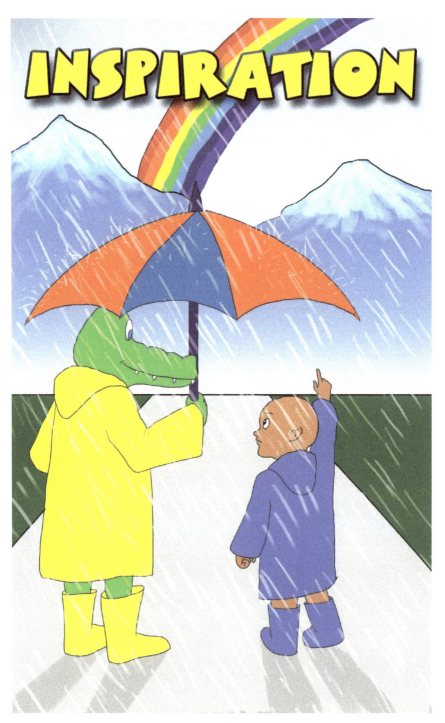

"I" is for inspiration;
it's the next one in line.
It helps me dream and helps pass the time.
It reminds me I do
what I dream and I choose.
It reminds me life's good,
and I've got nothing to lose.

Inspiration is that feeling I get
when I'm walking in rain and all soaking wet.
It's the moment in mind
when the light bulb turns on,
when all the doubt runs,
disappears, and is gone.

Inspiration is what you can find all around.
When you need it most,
it's right there to be found.
It's that feeling that tells you
to fight cancer; you'll win!
It's the feeling inside
that never lets you give in.

It's that feeling of believing
I will win that race;
no matter how tired,
I can keep up the pace.
I draw inspiration from whatever I do,
from whomever I know,
and those I love, too!

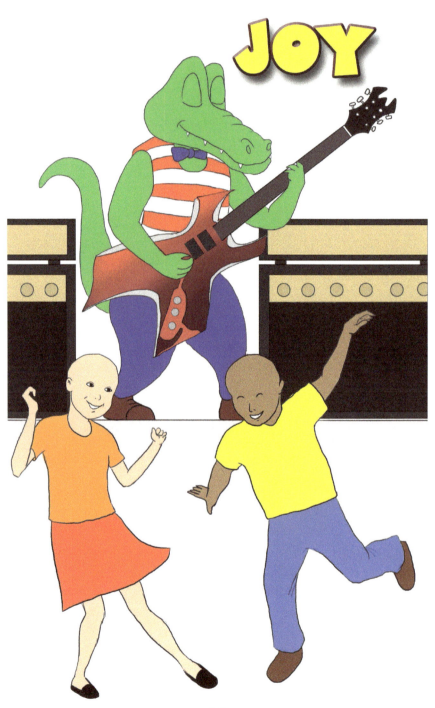

JOY

"J" is for joy, such a fun little word
that makes me feel light,
like the flight of a bird.
It's the feeling I get
when I play music and dance,
when I make a decision
or just take a chance.

It's that crazed happy feeling
when I hear some guitar,
when I sing in the shower
or the backseat of a car.
It's that feeling that reminds me
I'll always survive.
It's the feeling that proves
that I'm here, I'm alive!

Joy is something so small and so sweet;
it's me laughing hard
when you tickle my feet.
It touches my heart and soars in my head,
and even stays with me
as I sleep in my bed.

Joy is something that coaxes my smile.
It makes me relax like a kid for a while.
It helps me get through
the toughest of days.
It shows me I'm alive in so many ways.

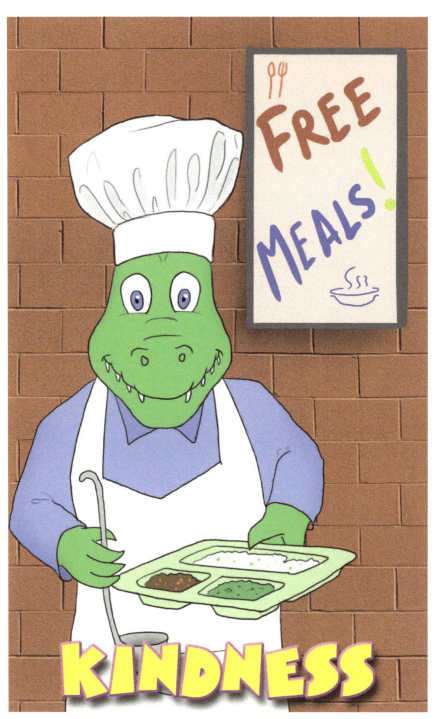

The ABC's of Surviving Cancer

"K" is for kindness, something I do or I say.
It's something I mention
when I stop and I pray.
It's something that makes me
feel happy and good,
and something I'd show everyone,
yes I would!

It's helping when someone
is crossing the street.
It's the smile I still give you
when you sing off beat.
It's the way you love me
even when you're mad,
and how you treat me
when I'm sick or I'm sad.

Kindness is something
that cannot bought.
It's something to show
and something that's taught.
It's lending a hand when someone's in need,
helping the homeless,
or some other good deed.

It's something to do that touches the heart,
and no matter the outcome
it's a very good start.
Kindness is something
that helps everyone heal.
Kindness is something that cancer can't steal.

LOVE

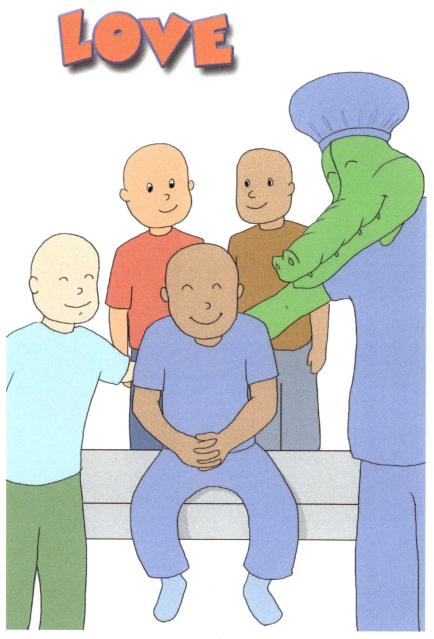

So the next letter is "L,"
and it stands for love.
It's such a blessing, it's sent from above.
It's something we're given
to make a great life,
and something for everyone,
not just husband and wife.

See, love can come from family or friends.
It can come in a word
or a gift someone sends.
It's a feeling that makes
me happy and strong,
and helps me keep faith
when life seems to go wrong.

Love is a bond between parent and child.
When we're older
it's a feeling all crazy and wild.
It's a smile, a touch, or a look on my face.
It's a cuddle, a story, or flowers in a vase.

Love is the reason I continue to fight.
Love lights my path
with the brightest of light.
It's the proof that reminds me
I'm never alone,
and a feeling I get
whether I'm young or all grown.

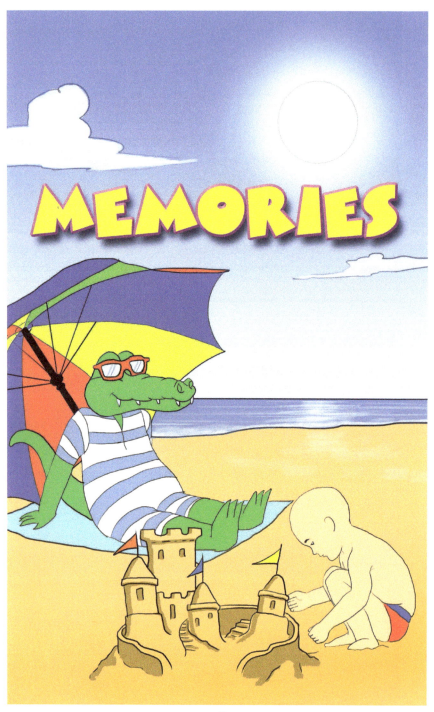

"M" is for memories.
They're quite a big deal.
They're thoughts of my family
eating a meal.
They're what I'll remember
when I'm all grown,
when I'm married with kids
and all on my own.

Memories remind me I have something to do.
They help me remember to say, "I love you."
I have memories of good things
like laughter and fun,
a day at the beach in the sand and the sun.

Memories are something I cannot deny,
like that look on your face
when I keep asking, "Why?"
I'll remember the ways
I made you so proud,
and the joy in your laughter
when I'm silly and loud.

Memories can be good or they can be bad.
They can make us feel happy
or make us quite sad,
but the great thing about
a memory, you see:
It's something that's mine
and lives inside me.

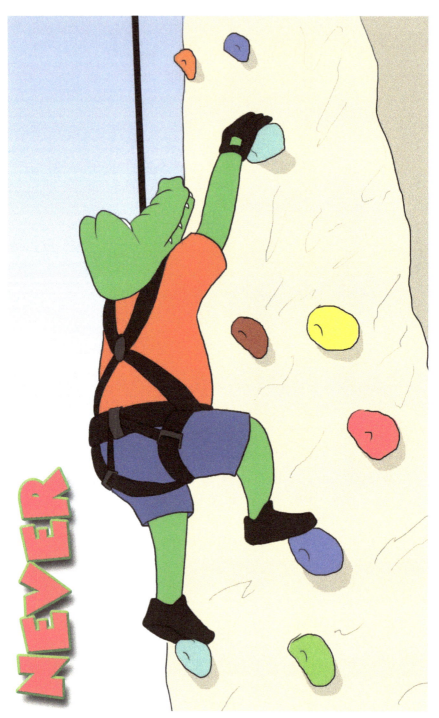

NEVER

The ABC's of Surviving Cancer

"**N**" is for never
and it's important, you'll see,
when I'm fighting the fire
of cancer in me.
See, it's very important I never give in.
I never give up; I'm determined to win.

I'll never admit or give in to defeat.
It's never okay for me to get beat.
See, there are things that cancer
can never take,
like a game of football
or a big birthday cake.

There's never a time
I won't laugh or have fun.
There's never a time
I'll give up and be done.
There's one thing you taught
from the time I was small:
When it comes to life, I give it my all.

So you don't forget, I'll say it again:
I never give up, and I never give in,
and no matter what,
on the darkest night,
remember I'll never stop,
I'll always fight!

OPTIMISTIC

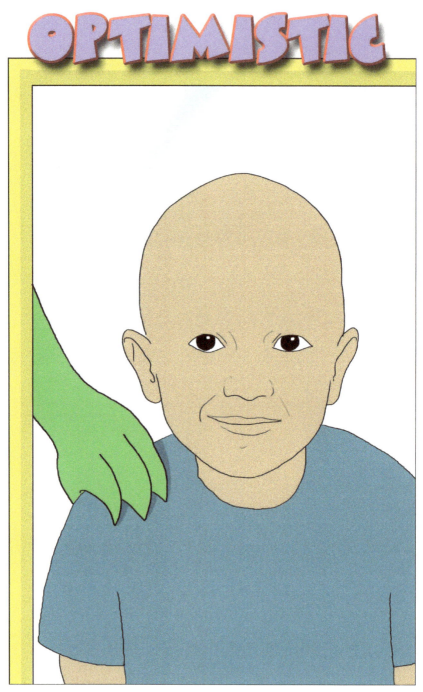

The ABC's of Surviving Cancer

Optimistic, is the word for "O."
It's something I am wherever I go.
It's that positive energy that lives inside,
and the idea of sun
when it's raining outside.

It's the word for me
that explains why I fight.
It's that thing inside
turning darkness to light.
It's the way I see life on a positive note
when I know I'll survive
even a sinking boat.

Being optimistic is what
I like and I choose.
I'll be happy and positive if I win or I lose.
My happy is something that can't be taken;
my positive ways
can't be stolen or shaken.

See, it's the light inside me
that cancer can't put out.
It's my positive energy
that gets rid of all doubt.
It's the feeling inside
that helps keeps me alive.
It's that driving force
that helps me survive.

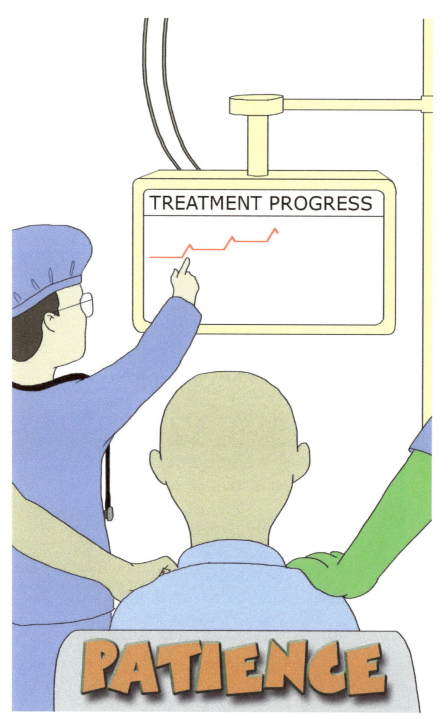

The ABC's of Surviving Cancer

"P" is for patience; it's the hardest for me.
It's those times that drag out
when I'm waiting to see.
It's those times when I think
the clock is what broke,
when I was expected to keep quiet,
but blew it and spoke.

Patience is something I'll learn as I grow.
It's not something I'm born with,
yet something I know.
Patience helps me when I want to get mad;
it helps me avoid anger
when I'm sick and I'm sad.

It reminds me that sometimes
I can't get my way.
I have to have patience,
even if I've waited all day.
It reminds me that no matter
how big or how small,
patience is important for one and for all.

I need to remember, I won't have to wait long.
I need to have patience;
I need to stay strong,
because patience is something
that I can sure use
when I'm young or I'm old
and waiting for news.

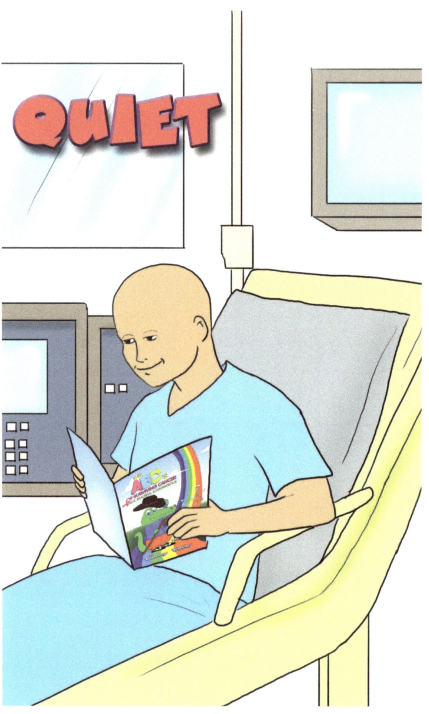

36

"Q" is for quiet, when I don't say a lot,
when I'm feeling sick or just got a shot.
It's one of the ways I focus and heal,
and for me being quiet
is quite a big deal.

Sometimes I sit and just read a book.
Sometimes I hang out
and watch someone else cook.
Sometimes I just need to quietly weep.
Sometimes when I'm quiet,
you won't hear a peep.

Sometimes the quiet can still my mind.
It can help me stay calm
and help me unwind.
It can make me feel rested,
feel well and quite ready,
even when my outside
is shaking and unsteady.

See, quiet is something I do pretty well;
I'll write and I'll read,
and I'll sit for a spell,
and then in an instant, the quiet is done,
and it's time to laugh,
be loud, and have fun.

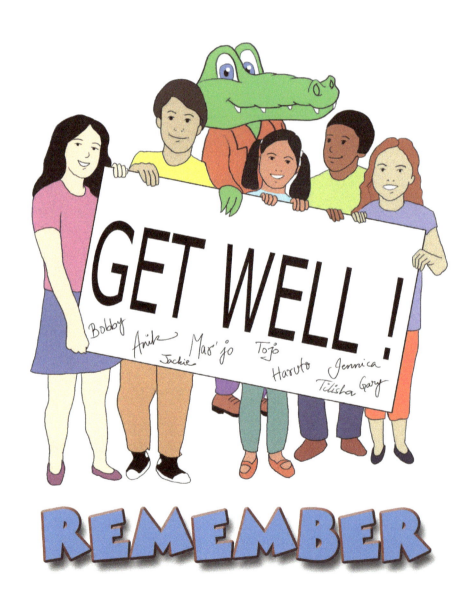

REMEMBER

The ABC's of Surviving Cancer

"R" is for remember, things I'll never forget,
like my first day at school
or the day we all met.
My friends came by,
and for a while they stayed.
We giggled and laughed
at the big card they made.

We all shared some stories,
good times from our past,
and agreed as we get older,
time seems to go fast.
It was great to remember
the things we've done.
I can't wait to feel better
so I can play and have fun.

They helped me remember
that I still need to smile.
They also reminded me I'm a kid for a while.
They proved once and for all I'm never alone,
and someday this will end,
and I'll get to go home.

They helped me remember
I'm brave and I'm strong.
They gave me memories to remember
when the days get long.
They helped me remember
things I thought I forgot.
They helped me remember
that I'm missed a lot!

STRENGTH

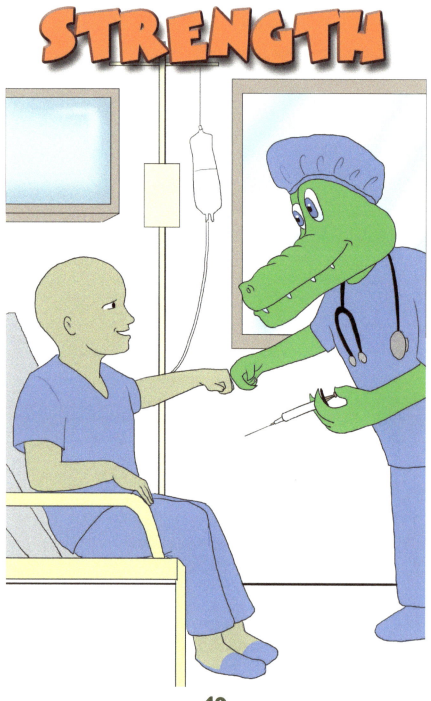

"S" is for strength, and the word says it all.
It's another that's helps me get up when I fall.
It's something inside me I pull out when I'm sick.
At my weakest moments, it's strength that I pick.

It's my strength others see
when I'm down and I smile,
when I'm getting my treatment,
and have to sit for a while.
My strength can be seen in so many ways,
it's my strength that shines through
on the darkest of days.

Strength is one of those actions I choose,
so in the weakest of moments, it's strength that I use.
That is what tells me, "You can fight this and win!"
It's my strength that reminds me,
"Never give up or give in!"

Always remember you'll find strength inside you,
and at the weakest of moments
it helps pull you through.
So just use your strength in good times and bad.
It's always with you whether you're happy or sad.

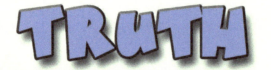

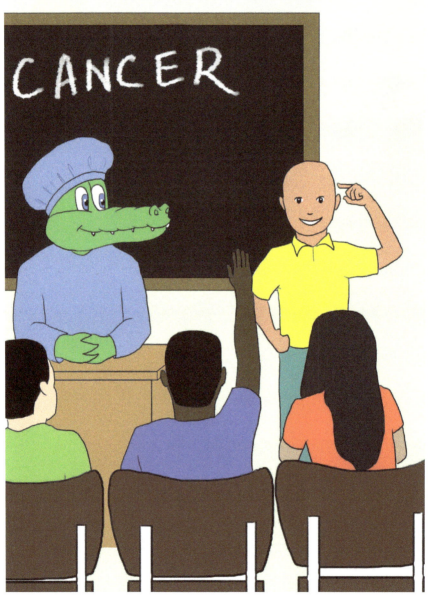

The ABC's of Surviving Cancer

"T" is for truth; I have cancer, you see.
It's not who I am; it's just an illness in me.
So if you're curious,
speak up and just say.
I'll tell you the truth;
all questions are okay.

I'm going to just say it:
"We must fight, we must win!"
I'll definitely tell you,
"Never give up or give in."
I'm going to remind you to always be true,
and that your optimism
is what gets you through.

You'll need lots of courage
to help in your fight,
but believe in your dreams;
they'll help you at night.
I'll remind you you're alive,
beautiful, and courageous,
and don't worry 'bout my cancer;
it's not contagious.

I'll tell you the truth
because I want you to see
the love and the joy
and the hope inside me.
I want you to know the ways I'll survive
and all that's in me that keeps me alive.

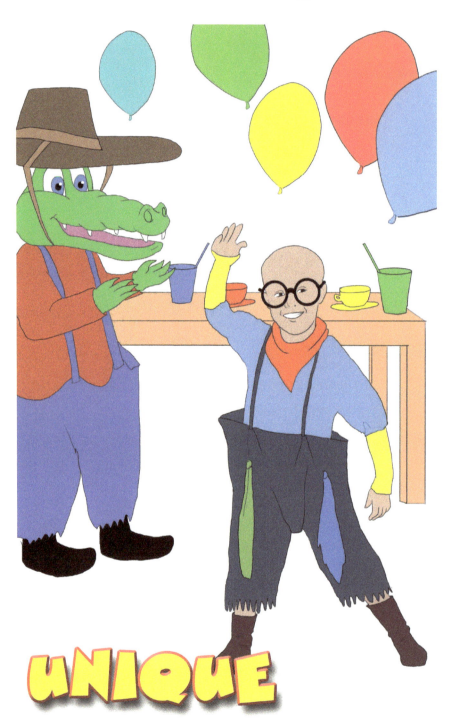

UNIQUE

"U" is for unique; that's what I'll be.
Cancer can't define what others will see.
I'll be funny and positive,
and I'll make you giggle.
I'll wear funny pants,
and I'll laugh and I'll wiggle.

I know fun is important
'cause it helps me heal,
and smiling affects how I act and I feel.
I want to make others feel happy and good.
I'd make everyone healthy
and smile, if I could.

See, I'm fun and unique
in my own special way.
I stay positive in all that I do and I say.
I know that no matter
what tomorrow brings,
what matters the most
is more than just things.

It's being one of a kind
in so many ways.
It's being myself in all of my days.
Knowing I'm special is what helps me cope.
It's that uniqueness inside
that gives me hope.

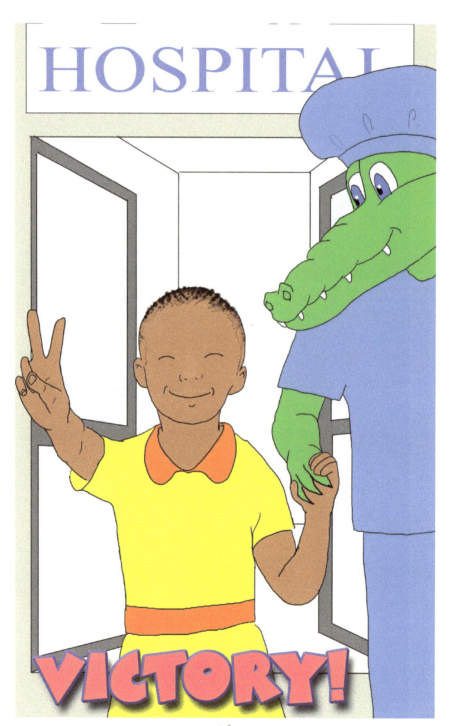

"V" is for victory;
I'm shouting, "Yes, I win!"
Because I never gave up,
and I never gave in.
I battled my illness and,
yes, I stayed strong,
even when I felt sick,
and the days grew long.

Victory is what's defined as success,
when things go my way,
and I'm definitely blessed.
I don't always win, and that's okay, too;
but I always achieve victory
in all that I do.

I try to find victory in whatever I face,
whether using my patience
or running a race;
and this time for me
it was a fight through tough days,
but still I found victory in so many ways.

Victory for me is different, you see.
It's each little goal as I fight cancer in me.
It's not just going home
when my treatment's all done,
it's that feeling of happiness
when I know I have won!

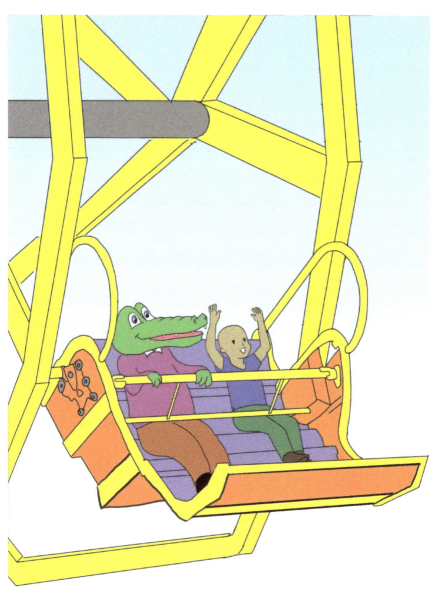

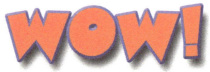

"W" is for "Wow!
Hey, I made it through!"
Now my days are so different,
I'm not sure what to do.
Maybe I'll visit the zoo or the park.
Maybe I'll stay out
from morning till dark.

Maybe I can ride a horse or a bike.
I guess I can do whatever I like.
An amusement park is tops on my list.
I plan on making up for all that I missed.

I'll ride the Ferris Wheel
straight to the top,
and way up there high
is right where we'll stop.
I know the view
is extremely outrageous,
and the smile on my face
will be completely contagious.

Wow! is how I know that I'll feel,
when I'm finally at home, eating a meal.
Wow! describes my every new action,
the feeling inside
of complete satisfaction!

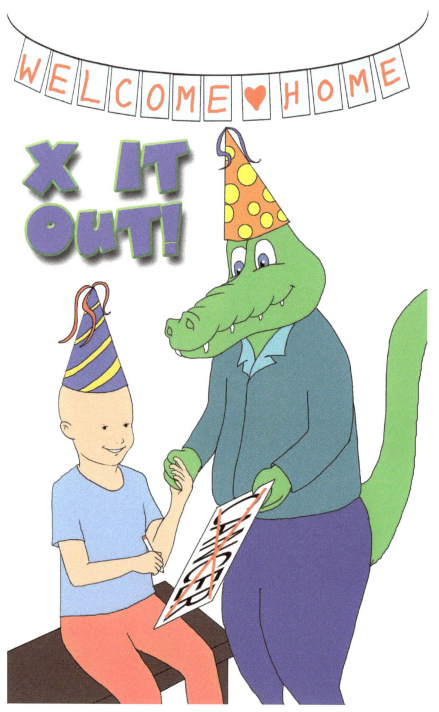

The ABC's of Surviving Cancer

So let's "X it out," the goal of the fight.
It's what we do to turn darkness to light.
An X next to healthy means that I'm good;
I fought my cancer as hard as I could.

I'll stay healthy and strong
and give it my best,
and celebrate the results
of each follow-up test.
I've X'd out my cancer
and fought this good fight;
I've stayed positive and strong,
so my future's quite bright.

X as a symbol sure gets marked a lot,
like on a treasure map
where X marks the spot.
On a computer you hit X
when you're finished and done.
On some video games,
it can mean that you won.

"X factor" is used to explain the unknown,
those mysteries in life
not explained on their own.
X on a calendar can mean the day's done.
On my calendar it means
I'm going home, and "I won!"

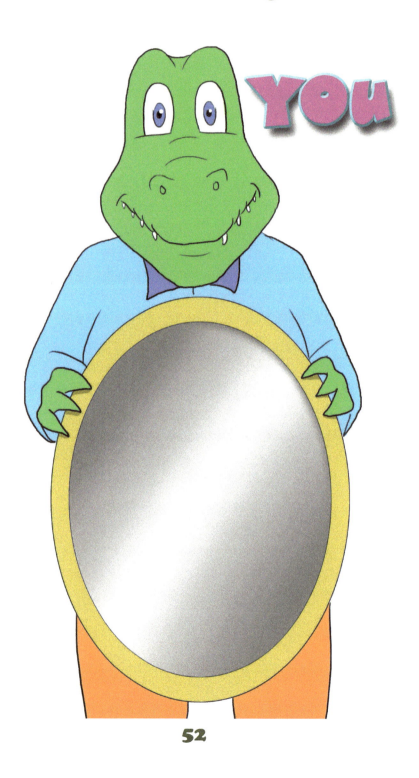

The ABC's of Surviving Cancer

You is the word for "Y."
It's the next letter in line.
It's by far the most important;
you'll see in good time.
It's the one that'll remind you:
This book is all about you,
the ways you can fight cancer,
and get yourself through.

So many things we dream,
and all that we can be,
are inspired by our lives
and each day that we see,
energy and courage will help you if you fall,
like love, joy, and kindness
for one and for all.

You are beautiful, courageous, and alive!
You know how to fight,
and what it takes to survive!
You'll be the one
showing others how you fight.
You will be the one
who turns darkness into light!

I believe that you know
love, joy, and how to dream.
You can define how to live
and what exactly life means.
If you look in the mirror, I think that you'll see
all that you are, and all you can be.

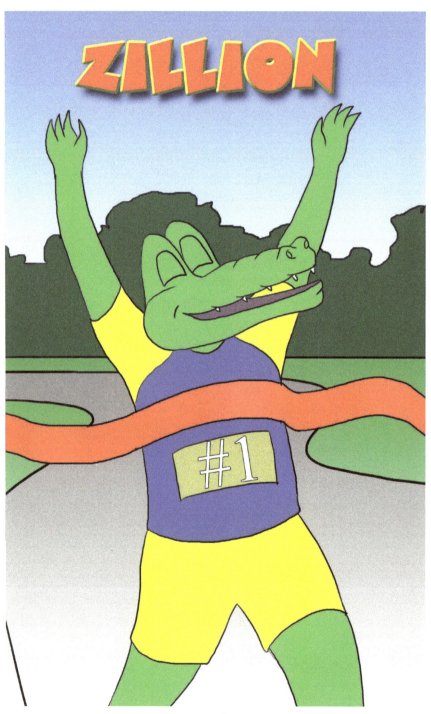

"Z" is for zillion; it's the last letter in line.
It's so very important,
you'll see in good time.
I can name many reasons
that I won this fight,
a zillion ways how
I turned darkness to light.

A zillion reasons
I never gave up or gave in,
a zillion ways I was going to win,
a zillion reasons I'll help you, too,
to discover the treasures inside of you.

A zillion days optimistic and strong,
and a zillion times
I proved cancer wrong.
I'm beautiful, courageous,
and have lots of hope,
and a zillion ways I'll guide you to cope.

I'll show you that although I may be small,
my joy, love, and strength
kept me standing tall.
I'll dream and I'll giggle,
and I'll help you see,
the zillions of ways...

I beat the cancer in me!

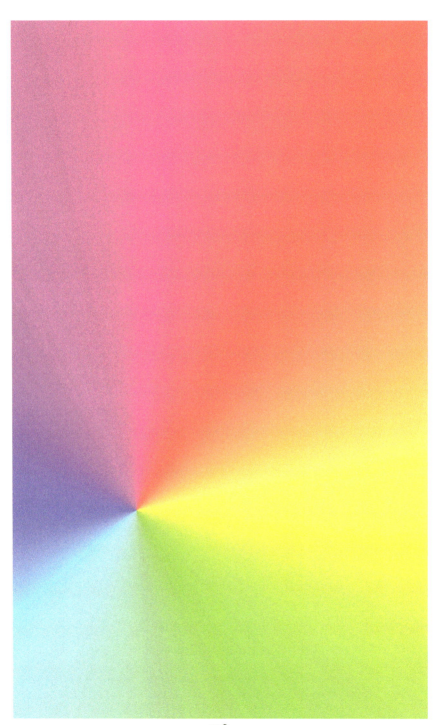

So if you have cancer
and are fighting the fight,
pull strength from within
and turn darkness to light.

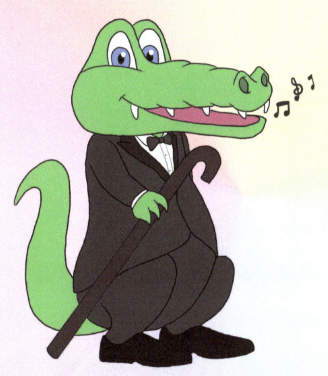

Never give up;
never give in
because beauty and courage
come from within.

Acknowledgements

I can't possibly name all the people who have helped and encouraged me with this project, but I have to single out a few:

I would like to thank the sponsors who made the book possible, people so dedicated to helping others they were willing to provide financial support to a project that speaks to kids and their loved ones. Notice their information at the back of the book, and be sure to support them back. You will never find a better group of caring people.

I am grateful for my daughters, Breanna and Jennica, who helped me endure the treatment, and who make every day of my life a joy. We went through this together, strengthening the bonds that will carry us through life. Now my granddaughters, Zoey and Sadie, are carrying on that tradition.

Thanks to MJ, my manager and the man in my life. You helped with every aspect of this project and made me believe in myself and what I could do for others. MJ also conceived the character of Cornelius!

I also want to acknowledge my parents, Mom Robbie and Dad Gary Howard, and my grandmother, Nellie. We lost Dad recently, so I'll miss all the ways he reminded me of who I am. Mom is always there for me. You worked hard to see this project to fruition, especially providing the art that inspired the images of Cornelius. Grandma Nellie has passed on, but she lives on in many ways, including the name of Cornelius, about whom she dreamed.

I will always be grateful to the countless medical people who helped me survive. I can't possibly name you all, but you are legion, the good-hearted and hard-working souls who pick us up and carry us when we need it most.

Thank you, Jackie Hendon, for helping me find the best possible publisher for my project.

Finally, I thank the good people at my publisher, Fresh Ink Group, who assembled the book, and who created the illustrations, the website, the promotional video on YouTube, and more. Ann Stewart is the master at book design who built all the files, including all the ebook editions. Beem Weeks is the social-media director who is helping me with promotion, including managing my new website. Anik did the beautiful illustrations of Cornelius. Mukesh built my website, which I am very proud of. Most of all, I want to thank Stephen Geez. You believed in me since the first moment I spoke with you about my dream of writing a book. You have encouraged me and even kicked me in the butt when I needed it. You have gone so far above and beyond for me there is no way I could ever thank you enough! I have been very blessed to have you as a publisher, editor, and inspiration.

About the Author

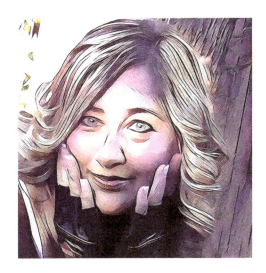

Now a mother and grandmother, Tammy Trover is a veteran and longtime cancer survivor who works for the Veterans Administration helping vets coordinate their medical benefits. She holds a B.S. in Criminal Justice, and is now working on her master's degree. A native of Maine, she lives in Denver, Colorado.

www.TammyTrover.com

Twitter: @TSTrover1
Facebook: Author Tammy Trover
Email: Contact@TammyTrover.com

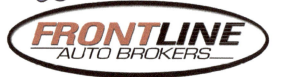
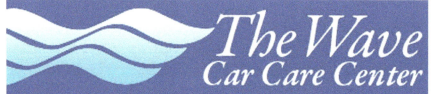
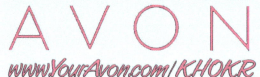

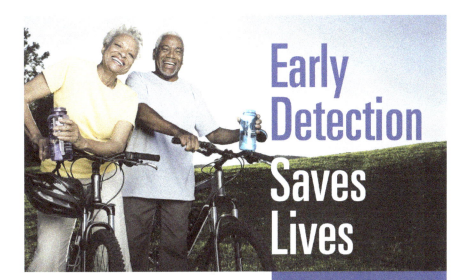

Early Detection Saves Lives

Colon cancer is the third leading cause of death in the United States, while **9 out of 10** cases can be prevented through early detection.

Over 50? Family History? Get Screened!

Direct Screening Available – Call Today!

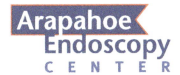

Arapahoe Endoscopy CENTER

1001 Southpark Dr. Littleton, CO 80120
Phone: 720-772-5550
Fax: 720-772-5551

 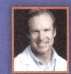

From top:
Bahri Bilir, MD
Nuray Gun, MD
James Rhee, MD
Andrzej Triebling, MD

From top:
Luke Evans, MD
Steven Lawrence, MD
Erik Springer, MD
Philip Sarges, MD

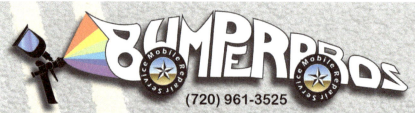

BUMPERPROS

Mobile Repair Service · Mobile Repair Service

(720) 961-3525

Making cars beautiful, one bumper at a time

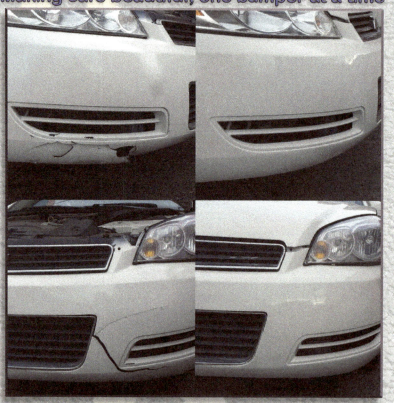

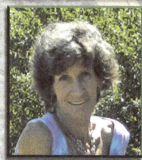

In honor of our own Loretta,

Alive, beautiful, and courageous,

A fighter who never gives up!

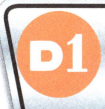
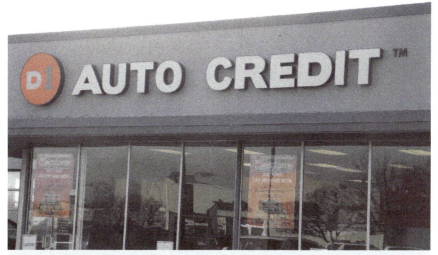

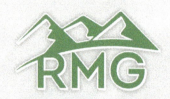

ROCKY MOUNTAIN
GASTROENTEROLOGY

Rocky Mountain Gastroenterology
Arapahoe Group
in Littleton

1001 Southpark Drive Littleton, CO 20120
303-722-8987

Bahri Bilir, MD

Nuray Gun, MD

James Rhee, MD

Erik Springer, MD

Luke Evans, MD

Steven Lawrence, MD

Philip Sarges, MD

Andrzej Triebling, MD

http://www.rockymountaingastro.com/locations/rmg-arapahoe-littleton

Talk to us about
Colon Cancer
Prevention & Screening

The Fresh Ink Group

Publishing
Free Memberships
Share & Read Free Stories, Essays, Articles
Free-Story Newsletter
Writing Contests

Books
E-books
Amazon Bookstore

Authors
Editors
Artists
Professionals
Publishing Services
Publisher Resources

Members' Websites
Members' Blogs
Social Media

www.FreshInkGroup.com

Email: info@FreshInkGroup.com

Twitter: @FreshInkGroup

Google+: Fresh Ink Group

Facebook.com/FreshInkGroup

LinkedIn: Fresh Ink Group

About.me/FreshInkGroup

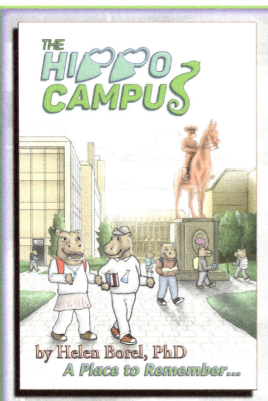

THE
HIPPO
CAMPUS

by Helen Borel, PhD
A Place to Remember...

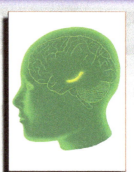

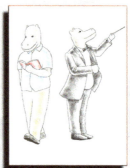

The Interactive Brain Book: Fun Learning for Science Lovers

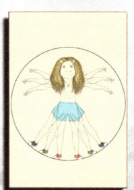

Fresh Ink Group
www.FreshInkGroup.com

Helen Borel, PhD
@BorelMedWriter

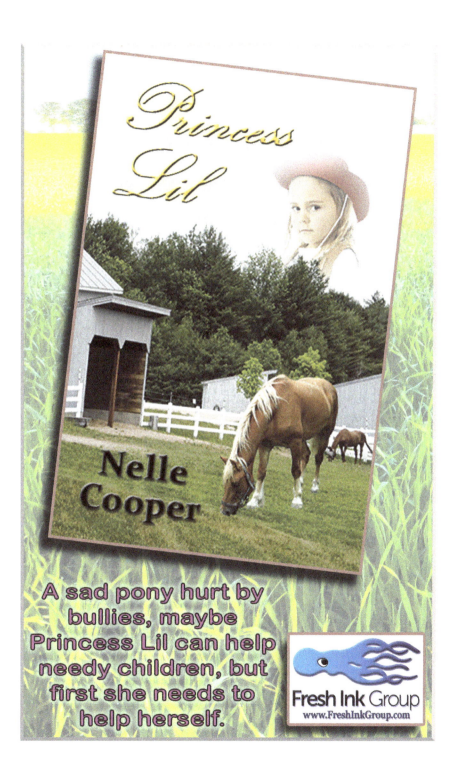

Princess Lil

Nelle Cooper

A sad pony hurt by bullies, maybe Princess Lil can help needy children, but first she needs to help herself.

Fresh Ink Group
www.FreshInkGroup.com

Lightning Source UK Ltd.
Milton Keynes UK
UKHW022002270219

338146UK00009B/249/P